**Ali Hassan**
**Guenther Kieninger**

# Primary Repair of Infected Pilonidal Cyst by Limberg Flap

Ali Hassan
Guenther Kieninger

# Primary Repair of Infected Pilonidal Cyst by Limberg Flap

LAP LAMBERT Academic Publishing

**Imprint**

Any brand names and product names mentioned in this book are subject to trademark, brand or patent protection and are trademarks or registered trademarks of their respective holders. The use of brand names, product names, common names, trade names, product descriptions etc. even without a particular marking in this work is in no way to be construed to mean that such names may be regarded as unrestricted in respect of trademark and brand protection legislation and could thus be used by anyone.

Cover image: www.ingimage.com

Publisher:
LAP LAMBERT Academic Publishing
is a trademark of
Dodo Books Indian Ocean Ltd. and OmniScriptum S.R.L publishing group

120 High Road, East Finchley, London, N2 9ED, United Kingdom
Str. Armeneasca 28/1, office 1, Chisinau MD-2012, Republic of Moldova, Europe
Managing Directors: Ieva Konstantinova, Victoria Ursu
info@omniscriptum.com

Printed at: see last page
**ISBN: 978-3-8473-3584-9**

# PRIMARY REPAIR OF INFECTED PILONIDAL CYST WITH LIMBERG FLAP

DR ALI HASSAN

Prof. Guenther Kieninger

## INTRODUCTION

Pilonidal Sinus or Pilonidal cyst is a common disease. When it gets  infected it becomes annoying for the patient and embarrassing for the  surgeon.Too many  medical terms were given to this disease .Some are still used such as Dermoid cyst; Sacral Dermoid, Sacrococcygeal cyst. They all  describe the anatomical location .According to the Consensus of the German society for Proctologic surgeons and Dermatologists 2007 – 2008 only pilonidal sinus should be used for this disease, because the  other synonyma might be misleading.

We believe, inspite of the consensus, that the term **Pilonidal cyst** correct to describe the formation in the Sacrococcygeal area, while  Pilonidal Sinus describes only the tract through which the pus or  discharge are evacuating. Both entities are differently coded in I.c.d: Pilonidal cyst with abscess is coded L05-01 while Pilonidal Sinus with abscess is L05-02.

In this book we will be using both terms, mainly pilonidal cyst, because it gives a better understanding for the disease.

The treatment of the infected pilonidal cyst is always a surgical. Too many surgical procedures have been described. None till now has proven itself to be a Gold standard.

The above mentioned German Consensus stated that excision of Pilonidal Cyst and Primary Repair are justified only in non infected cases (or in chronic case). We will discuss in this book our experience in applying the Limberg technique in **infected** cases and will propose it as a gold standard for the treatment of Pilonidal cyst disease.

# PART I

# LIMBERG:

He is Prof. Alexander Alexandrovisc  Limberg (1894). A Soviet (Russian) Surgeon and Stomatologist, who worked as Maxillofacial Surgeon at Leningrade Institute  for Traumatology and Orthopedics. Prof. A. A. Limberg developed a number of

methods of taking ,transplanting and using pedicle grafts for facial defects, and was 1948 awarded the State Price of USSR for his monograph:""The Mathematical Basis of Local Plastic Surgery on the surface of human body"" .

The first paper  in the subject was published 1928. Only in 1963, Thomas Gibson from Glascow published the first paper in English in "Modern trends in Plastic Surgery"Where , for the first time ,Limberg flap was mentioned in relation

with the Pilonidal Cyst.

The **Limberg flap** is a rhomboid flap, basically a parallelogram with 2

angles, 60º and 120º which of course can be slightly modified

according to the shape of the lesion.

The flap was primary meant to close the defects in the face after

basal cell carcinoma or melanoma surgery.

The main importance of the flap lies in the fact that the defect is

filled with good vascularized tissue of the same thickness and color.

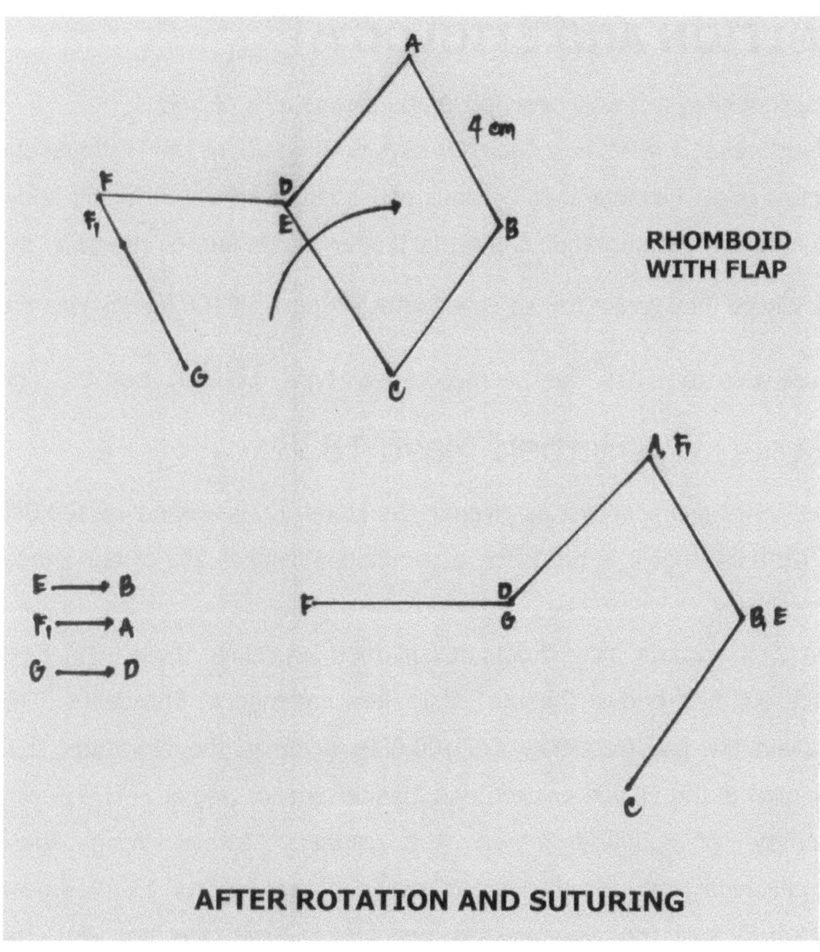

A
4 cm
F
F1
D
E
B
G
C
RHOMBOID
WITH FLAP
E → B
F1 → A
G → D
A F1
D
G
F
B E
C
AFTER ROTATION AND SUTURING

# DEFINITION AND ETIOLOGY:

The term pilonidal cyst is only descriptive and means nest of hair

*(pilus= hair; nidus = nest from Latin).* It says nothing about the Histiogenetic or Etiological origin.Pilonidal cyst or sinus can occur everywhere in the body. They are found in the suprapubic area, in Barber hands and of course in the umbilicus where they cause the so called infected navel. **Hodges** was the first to use this term for the Sacrococcygeal type **1880,** but the first description goes back to **Herbert Mayo 1833**.

The frequency of pilonidal cyst as given in the literature, is around 25/100,000 people.  We think that it is much more common. It makes 2% of our annual operation registry.

PILONIDA CYST occurs more frequently in men especially those who have much hairs on their bodies (hirsute), it is  less common in Europeans. This might explain the low frequency (25/100.000) given in the literature. It is more common in the Middle Eastern and Mediterranean  region. (This is why the majority of publication on this subject comes from those countries).Pilonidal sinus usually occurs between the ages of 15-34, (mean age 24 years) their development  is uncommon after the age 40! The youngest of our patients is a 14 years old girl. The oldest a 45 years old Diabetic man. Frequency Male / Female is in the range of 80/20.

The **Etiology** of Pilonidal Sinus is still debatable. It was believed For long time to be of congenital origin, as imperfect separation of the ectodermal and mesodermal layers during embryonic development.

Now a days pilonidal cyst is generaly considered to be an acquired disease as hairs perforate into subcutaneous layer especially byprofessionals with long time sitting.

During World War II nearly 80,000 soldiers developed this disease.Pilonidal Cyst was then given the name **Jeep drivers disease**. We have good reasons to adopt the acquired theory: Young men, intergluteal cleft, bad hygiene, sweating and, of course, adipositas are all conditions facilitating the hair to perforate in to the subcutaneous area.But on the other hand we have some reasons for the inborn theory: Young girls deep epithelial cover with contact to the <u>Sacrococcygeal fascia.</u>What ever the etiology is the treatment is the same, and so the discussion of being acquired or inborn is only of academic

interest.We can consider that pilonidal sinus is an acquired disease with congenital predisposition. Its development depends on multiplicity of factors. It starts with the hair perforating through the skin deep in the subcutaneous fat resulting in a foreign body granuloma, which can remain for life long without any symptoms **(Asymptomatic form)**. Or it can gets infected, leading to an abscess, chronic or acute **(symptomatic form)**.

# DIAGNOSIS.

It is very easy to diagnose a symptomatic Pilonidal Sinus. Pain, swelling, redness and eventually discharge from the sinus pits in the intergluteal fold are seen by simple inspection. No special imaging techniques  are necessary (CT scan, MRI etc).Perianal abscess or Fistulating Crohns Disease should be Considered as differential diagnosis. The anatomical location facilitates the diagnosis eliminating any confusion.

# Symptoms.

As we mentioned previously, Pilonidal sinuses can remain "Calm" for life not causing any symptoms. It is than called <u>Asymptomatic</u> ,not needing any therapy. It is diagnosed only by the presence of some pits in the intergluteal fold.

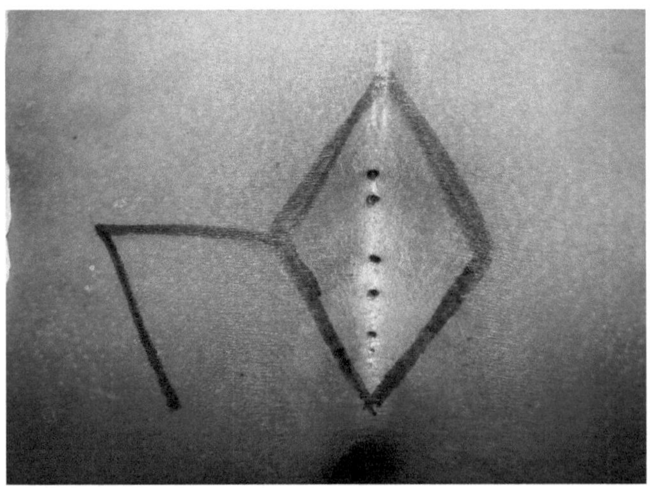

When the pilonidal cyst gets infected it becomes <u>Symptomatic like any abscess</u> either <u>acute </u>or <u>chronic</u>  (50/50).

Acute Pilonidal cyst abscess is very painful characterized by swelling, redness and pain in the midline or slightly lateral, fever and chills might be also present. Malignant degeneration after long term persistence is possible. Davis et al found till 1966 around 40 cases in the literature most of them epithelial carcinoma.

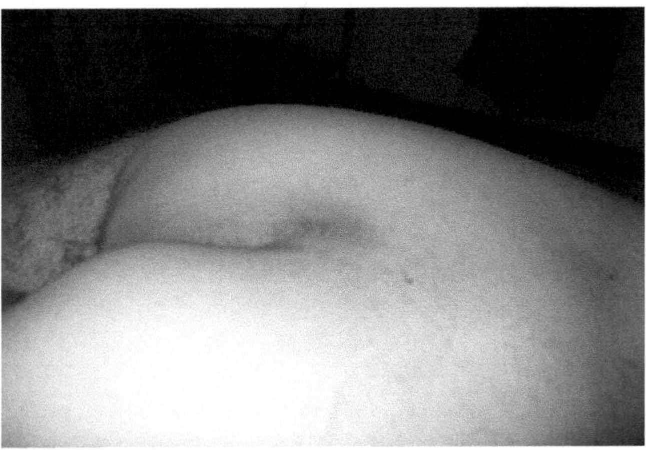

# Treatment.

<u>Asymptomatic</u> pilonidal sinus does not need any further treatment. The treatment of the symptomatic pilonidal sinus is always a surgical one. There are many methods described for the treatment of the pilonidal sinus disease, but none of them has been accepted till now as an optimal modality.Pilonidal sinus is not considered to be a major problem in terms of the surgical techniques. However considering the age group it mainly affects (young adults) it presents a serious condition that can cause a significant reduction in

labor and disruption of the educational process in the community. The simplest way to treat a pilonidal sinus abscess is incision and evacuation of the pus. The procedure can be done as out patient under local anesthesia. But the patient has to come later for definitive treatment as a cold
case. In general we can say that there are 3 options for the surgical
treatment of Pilonidal Cyst:

# 1.    Total excision leaving the wound open for secondary healing.

# 2.    Total excision and primary closure.

# 3.    Plastic repair

Each of the methods has advantages and inconvenient:
1. Total excision and secondary healing.
The advantage of this method is the short time of surgery and it can be done, as day case surgery.The advantage weigh only a little compared with the major inconvenient of very long healing period and frequent  dressing, a  reduced labor  time and  recurrence rate  20-50%.
2. Total excision with direct primary closure.
This method is accompanied with high rate of wound infection  and dehiscence and  over 50% recurrence rate.  It is applied only in chronic infection.
3. Total excision with plastic repair. Plastic procedure have a major advantage compared with the primary direct closure.

**Those advantages are:**

- Short duration of the hospitalization from 1-4 days
according to the policy  of the surgeon
- Quick healing time 14-21 days
- Very low risk of wound infection
- And very low recurrence rate less than 1%

Several plastic procedures have been described, the most important among them are Karidakys , Bascom, Z-plasty, X-Y, Marsupialization and of course the Limberg flap.

A comparison of the different procedures in terms of recurrence is shown in table 7.

The **Limberg Flap** now a days is generally adopted as method of choice in Chronic cases (German Consensus 2007-2008).It's superiority to other methods
is evident. the recurrence rate is less than 1%.

**The treatment goal of Pilonidal Sinus should aim to:**
- Short healing period
- Short hospitalization
- Quick recovery to work
- Reduce risk of infection
- Reduce risk of recurrence
- Good cosmetic results.

**To achieve this goal, the surgery should reach:**
- A tension free suturing
- Flattening of the intergluteal fold
- Avoid midline incision and shifting the suture line off midline

- Reduce recurrence
- Reduce vacuum effect
- Filling the cavity by similar tissue and same color

According to our experience , all these conditions are granted only by the **Limberg Flap.**

The new, and different ,in our experience is that we apply it in infected pilonidal cyst disease with excellent results as we will  show in the last chapter.

*Figure 1:*

**Few quick reminders**

- Pilos (hair)  Nidus (nest)
- First described 1833-Mayo
- Males: over 80%
- Mean age 24 years(rare over 45)
- 25 cases /100.000

*Figure 2:*

**<u>Pathophysiology</u>**

- **Congenital** – imperfect separation of the ectodermal and mesodermal layers during embryonic development.
- **Acquired** -  hair introduced from outside "jeep disease" (cleft, recurrence, giant cell, no hair follicle)
- **Mixed**

*Figure 3:*

**Presentation**

- **Asymptomatic** – Just midline pits in presacral area (Intergluteal cleft )
- **Symptomatic**
  o Acute abscess
  o Chronic sinus/es

*Figure 4:*

## Treatment Modalities

### Primary Definitive Treatment

A-   EXCISION + OPEN Secondary healing.

- 8-12 weeks, daily dressing
- Annoying to patient and doctor
- High recurrence rate 19%

*Figure 5:*

### Acute abscess

- **Incision and drainage**
- Advantage: local anesthesia, OPD
- Disadvantage: a second operation
- **Or primary definitive treatment**

*Figure 6:*

## Treatment Modalities

### Primary definitive treatment

B-   Excision and Primary Closure

1. Direct closure

2.ADAPTATION (THOMPSON)

3.Marsupilaization

4.Karidakys

5.Bascom

6.Flap procedures

✓ Z-plasty

✓ V-Y advanced flap

✓ **Limberg Flap**

*Figure 7:*

**Some data from the literature**

1. Heal by sec. intention 387 cases; follow up till 20 years; recurrence 19%

2. Marsupilalization 204 case; follow up 6 years; recurrence 6%

3. Excision + Primary closure 1129 case; follow up not mentioned recurrence  16%

4. Karydakys 6545 case; follow up 20 years; recurrence less than  1%

5. Bascom:218 patients; recurrence 10%

*Figure 8:*

**Randomized studies Limberg flap** (5 publications)

|  | Total Number | Infection/ Wound Dehiscence | Mean Hosp. Stay | Return To work | Recurrence | Numbness |
|---|---|---|---|---|---|---|
| Mean! | ➢ 1300 | 0-6% 1.2% studies | 6 hrs to 4.5 days | 8-17 days | 0-5% 1% | 10-19% |

*Figure 9:*

**Goal of treatment**

- Short healing
- Short hospitalization
- Quick recovery to work
- Reduce risk of infection
- Reduce risk of recurrence
- Good cosmetic result

*Figure 10:*

**TO ACHIEVE THIS GOAL TREATMENT SHOULD AIM TO:**

- Tension free primary closure
- Flattening of the intergluteal cleft
- Avoid midline incision and shift the suture line off midline.
- Reducing recurrence
- Reduce vacuum effect (Haematomas, Seromas and infection)  by adequately filling the cavity.

*Figure 11*

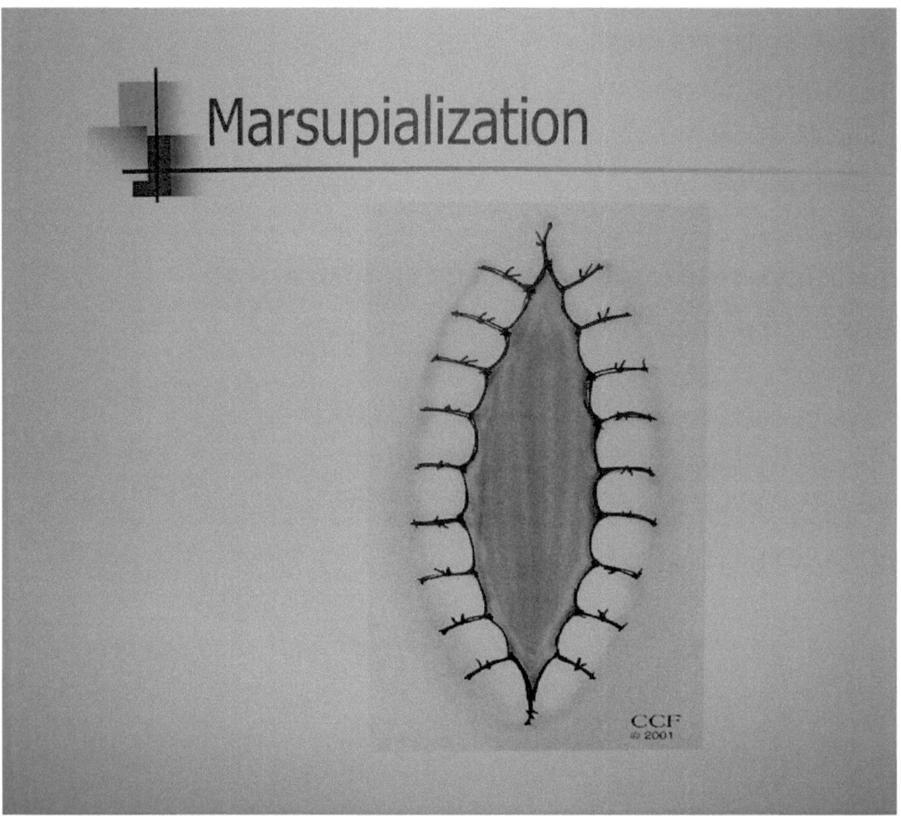

*Figure 12*

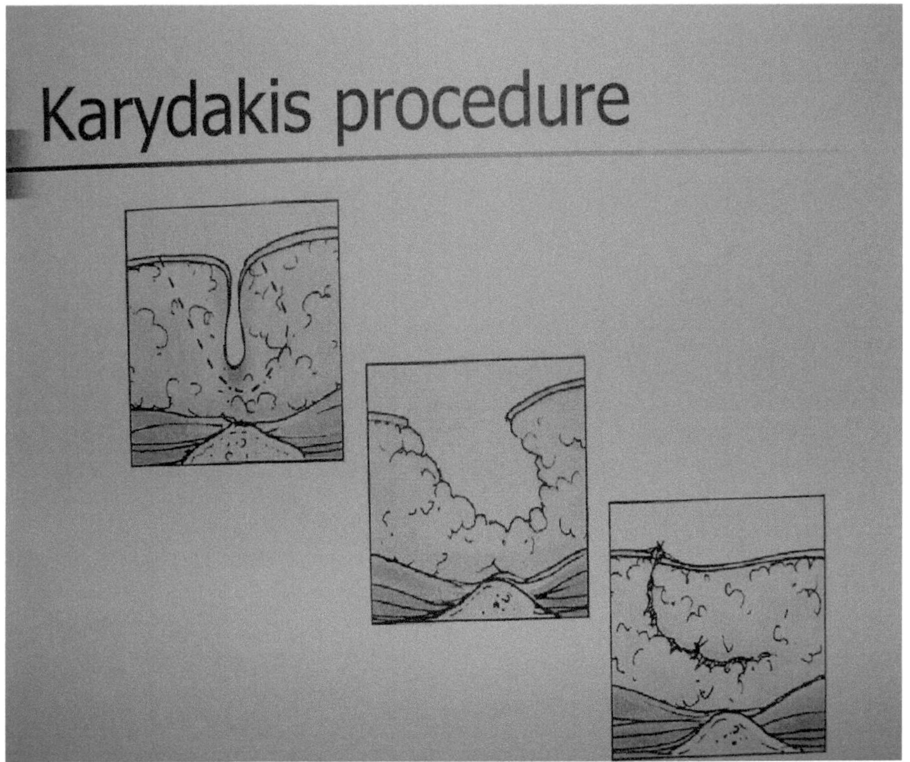

Figure 13

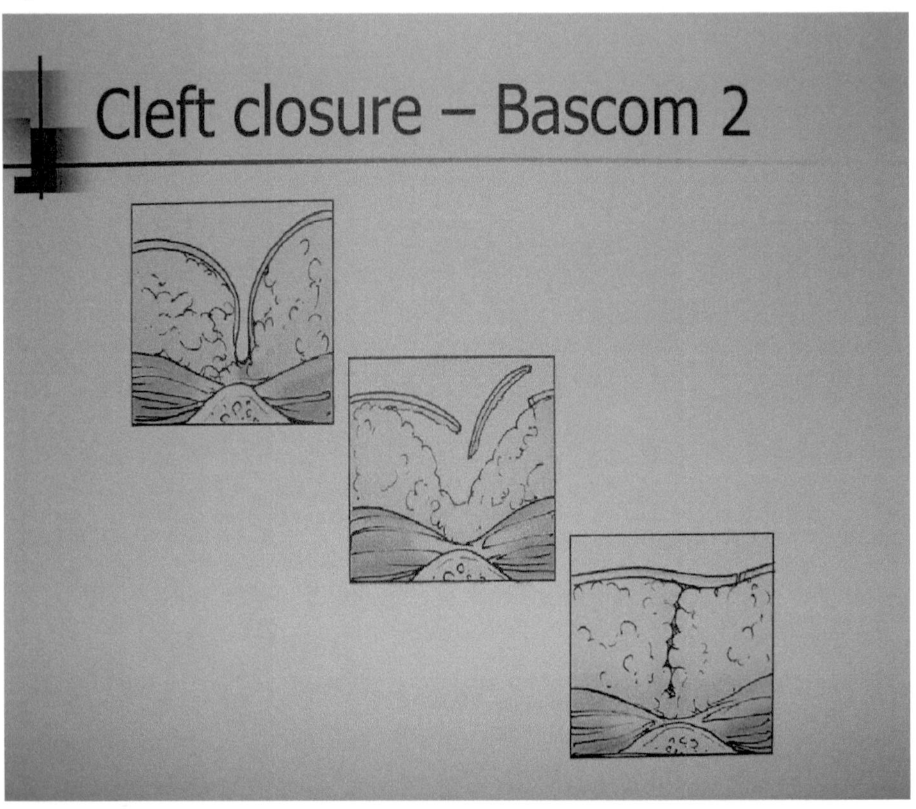
Cleft closure – Bascom 2

Figure 14

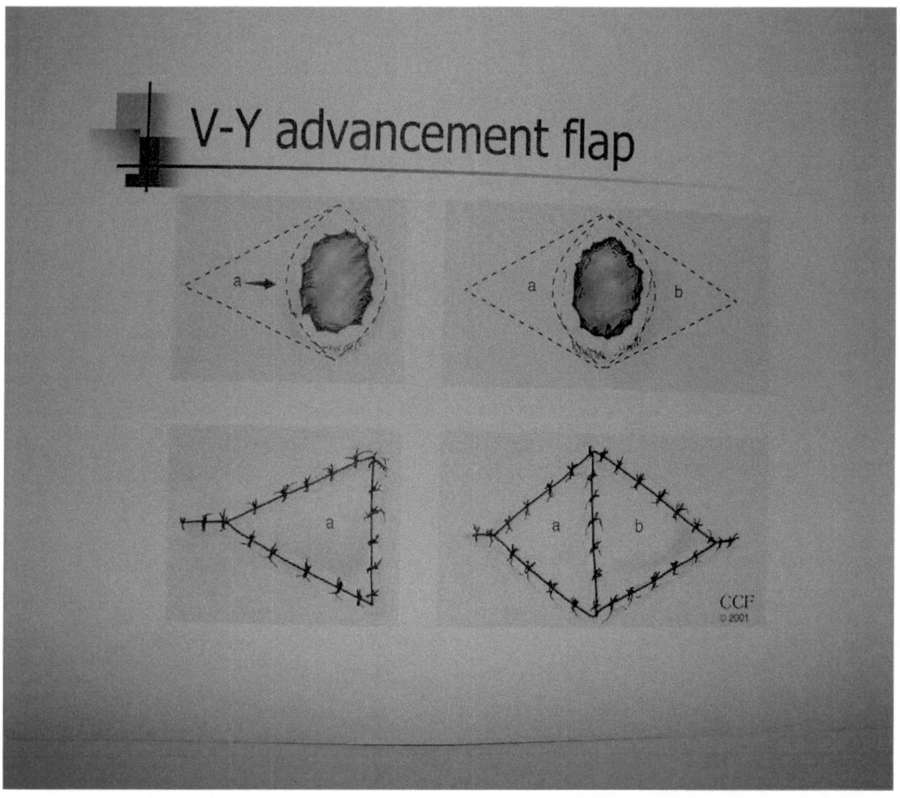
V-Y advancement flap
a
a
b
a
a
b
CCF
© 2001

*Figure 15*

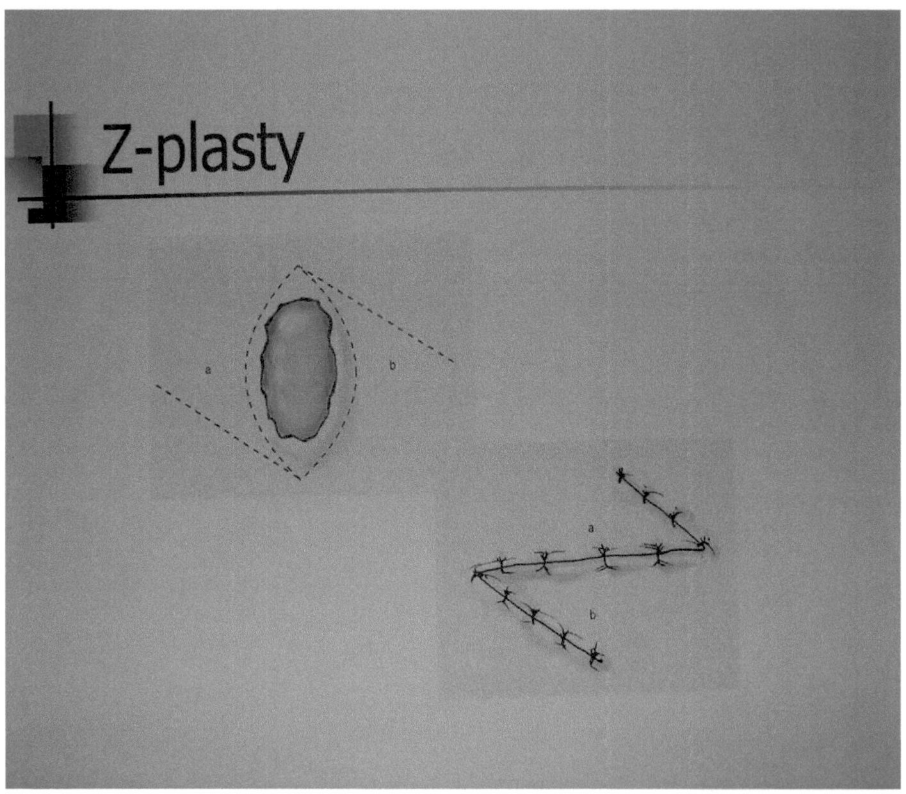

*Figure 16*

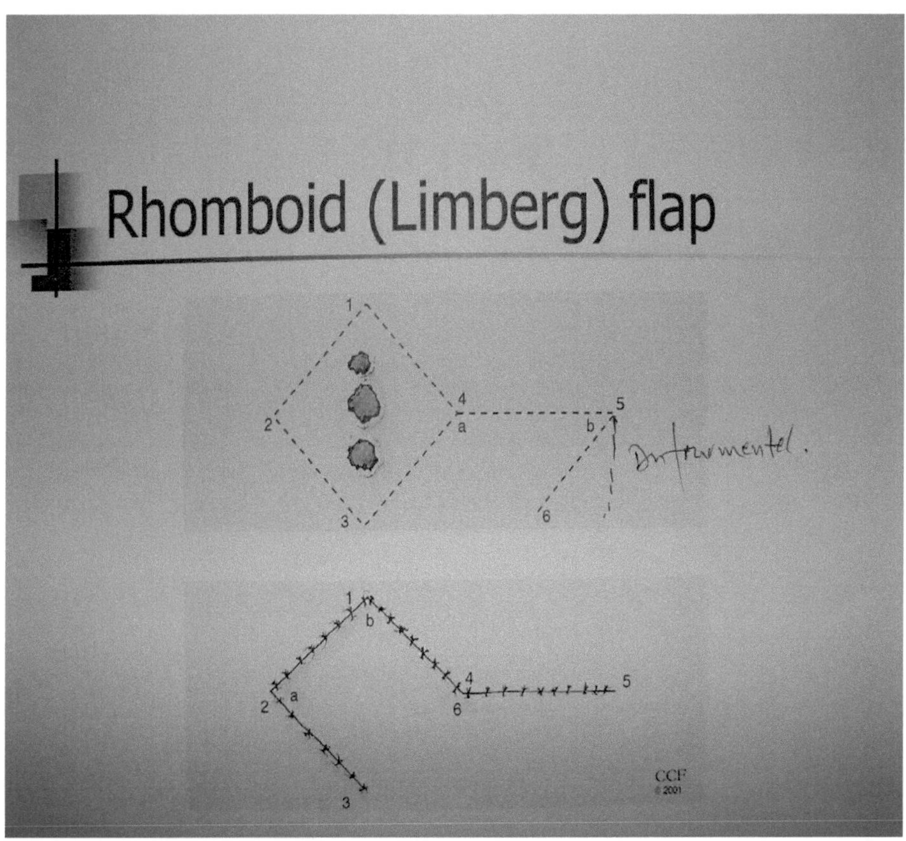

# PART II

# TREATMENT MODALITIES

## Comparison between the different techniques.

Pubmed shows for the last two years more than 1200 publications on pilonidal cyst disease. We have choosen some of these publications, dealing with surgical procedures used all over the world as a comparative work.

# 1. Open wound or midline closure

- **Lesianieks I, Furst A** from Surgical Clinic and Polyclinic of the University Regensburg, Germany published in "Der  Chirurg" 2003 an article "Pilonidal sinus" on a total of 73 patients. They stated that **midline closure** is associated with a **high recurrence rate** of 42%. They suggested that alternative operative techniques, creating a lateral wound and various skin flap procedures may be alternatives. "We are in process of **changing our treatment strategy for patients suffering** from pilonidal sinus" they said .

- . **De Parades V, Bouchard D, et al**published in  J.Vise Surg 2003 an article on pilonidal sinus disease. They stated that **excision is the standard definitive treatment**, but the choice of wide versus limited excision depends on the school of thought. The widespread practice in France is to leave the wound open, relying on postoperative healing by secondary intention. This technique has a low rate of recurrence, but the disadvantages are requirement of local nursing care and prolonged healing process, usually associated with a temporary, but prolonged cessation of activity.

"Primary wound closure techniques are less restrictive, but their recurrence rate is probably higher. A direct midline suture is best after a small excision, but for a more extended wound, plastic reconstruction techniques are preferred" they say.

■ **Fitzpatrick EB et al.** in Ann Surg 2013 did a retrospective cohort

analysis of operative therapy for pilonidal disease (PD) in a military population. **Results**: A total of 151 patients with PD were identified, who underwent excision (45.7%), excision with primary closure (29.8%), and incision and drainage (24.5%). Over all recurrence and morbidity rates were 37.2% and 34.4% respectively. Incision and drainage was associated with high recurrence rates >50%, and excision with primary closure was associated with increased complications .

- **Mc Callum IJ et al**. analysed 18 trials (N=1573) from Cochrane register of controlled trials (BMJ 2008 April), **comparing open healing with primary closure**. They found following results : Healing time was faster after primary closure, although data were unsuitable for aggregation. Rates of surgical site infection did not differ; recurrence was less likely to occur after open healing. Six trials compared surgical closure methods (midline versus off – midline). Wounds took longer to heal after midline closure than after off-midline closure (mean difference 5.4 days), rate of infection  and risk of recurrence were higher.

The **conclusion** was that wounds heal faster after
primary closure   than after open healing but at the expense of increased risk
of recurrence. Benefits were clearly shown with off- midline closure compared
with midline closure.**Off-midline closure should become standard
management for pilonidal sinus when  closure is the desired surgical
option.**


# 2. Karydakis

- **Horwood J, et al**. compared primary closure **Karydakis off-midline versus Limberg flap** in a meta analysis of randomized controlled trials (Colorectal Disease 2013): 641 patients in six studies were included. Rhomboid flap excision demonstrated a trend towards less disease recurrence (P=0.07), lower infection  (P=0.001) and dehiscence rate (P=0.01). However, no significant difference was found for pain scores, hospital stay or return to work.

They concluded that the currently published literature **supports the use of the rhomboid flap excision and the Limberg flap repair procedures over primary midline suture techniques for the elective management of primary pilonidal disease**.

- **Kamilyidiz M. et al.** published in  Scientific World   Journal 2013 an article on Karydakis flap procedure performed in  157 patients, stating that the **Karydakis procedure is one of the most  frequently used asymmetric flap techniques in the treatment of sacrococcygeal pilonidal sinus disease**.

This technique was  described by **Karydakis in 1973,** and         recurrence rates were reported to be < 1%. One of the significant     advantages of   the Karydakis  procedure is that it provides early return to daily activities in the postoperative period. While this period was reported to be 3-4 weeks using the primary midline closure technique, it was 12.4-20 days using the Karydakis method. The time elapse of returning to daily activities was 15 days in the current study. In addition, the postoperative patient satisfaction rate appears to be high with the Karydakis procedure.

**Can et al.**.reported that the degree of satisfaction was excellent in 70.8% of patients in their study. In the current study the patient satisfaction rate was 91.06%.

**The Karydakis flap procedure is a safe treatment alternative for the surgical treatment of sacrococcygeal pilonidal sinus disease because of associated low complication rate, short length of hospital stay and healing duration, and high patient satisfaction rate.**

# 3. V-Y and Limberg flap

In a study published 2013 in the J Korean Surg Soc, **Alfintoprak F, Dikiciere E et al**. from the Sakarya University, Turkey compared the results of 176 patients where  Limberg flap  or V-Y techniques were applied and they found that early postoperative and long term results of the Limberg flap and V-Y flap techniques were similar **but the resumption of daily activities at work was achieved later in patients undergoing the V-Y flap compared with the Limberg flap technique**. Patients' employment (or position in working life) must be considered when determining the most appropriate surgical technique.

# 4. Limberg flap

**Daphanc et al**. from the University of Kirikkele, Turkey(Dis Colon Rectum, 2004) reported the results of 147 male patients treated with Limberg flap in a soldier's hospital. They found that no major anesthetic or wound complication occured. Three patients (2 %)) developed a seroma (with negative culture) and six patients (4.1 %) had a partial wound detachment. Patients returned to full activity on the 10. − 25. postoperative day (mean 18.8). Patients were followed from 1 to 40  months. Seven patients (4.8 percent) had a recurrence. **They concluded that the Limberg flap procedure is an easy     and effective technique. Patient  comfort, quick healing time, early return to full activity, and low complication and recurrence rates are the important advantages of this procedure.**


# 5. Open healing versus Limberg

To compare the outcome of open excision and secondary healing with Rhomboid excision and Limberg flap in the management of pilonidal sinus disease, **J Amal et al**. from Liaquat University Hospital in Pakistan performed a prospective, analytical comparative study using a randomized controlled trial. In a total of 49 patients, who either underwent open excision and secondary healing (group A: 25 patients) or rhomboid excision and Limberg flap (group B:24  patients), were enrolled in the study. Duration of operation, postoperative pain, duration of hospital stay, postoperative complications, and time to recurrence were noted.

**Results:** Duration of operation was longer in group B patients   but pain perception was markedly reduced in this group. Total hospitalization period was shorter in patients in group B  and so was the time for complete healing of the wound . The recurrence rate was also significantly lower in patients who underwent Limberg rotation flap .

**Their conclusion: the Limberg flap is advantageous over simple excision and secondary healing in the management of pilonidal sinus.**

**Mentes BB et al**. (Surg Today 2004) analyzed the well documented records of 238 patients with sacrococcygeal pilonidal sinus who underwent wide excision with a Limberg transposition flap and were followed up for more than 1 year postoperatively. After the first 40 operations they modified the flap reconstruction by tailoring the rhomboid excision asymmetrically to place the lower pole of the flap 1-2 cm lateral to the midline. Wound infection rates, hospitalization time, time required for free mobilization, and recurrence rates were recorded.

**Conclusions:** The results provide further evidence that wide excision with Limberg transposition flap reconstruction is an effective surgical method for primary or recurrent pilonidal sinus, associated  with a low complication rate, short hospitalization and disability, and low recurrence rate. A modification of the technique was devised to further enhance wound healing and reduce the risk of recurrence.

# 6. V-Y versus Limberg

**Alfintoprak F,  Dikicier E, Aslan Y et al.** published in the J Korean Surg Soc 2013 a study investigating the results of their 176 patients operated with

Limberg flap, primary closure or V-Y flap. **They came to following conclusions:**

**A.** Although the primary closure method is known to result in a rapid recovery with a rapid resumption of daily activities, high complication and recurrence rates have been reported. The reasons for the negative results of the primary closure method are the incision scar in the midline, the inability to flatten the natal cleft, and the tissue tension. Various techniques have been described that attempt to eliminate the factors that cause these negative results of primary closure, resulting in lower recurrence rates.

**B.** Many factors (such as primary or recurrent disease, length of sinuses, defect size, patient preference, surgeon experience) are effective on flap technique selection. In this study was found that the early postoperative and long term results of the Limberg flap and V-Y techniques were similar, however, the V-Y technique had a longer resumption period of daily activities at work compared with Limberg technique. Therefore, we think that the patient's employment (or position in working life) should also be considered when determining which technique to use.

**Turfale AD et al.** published in the India J Surg 2012 an article comparing elliptical excision with midline primary closure versus Limberg flap in a prospective randomized study of 80 patients. They found that the parameters in which the two techniques were found to differ significantly were work-off period, immediate postoperative complications profile and recurrence rates. Rhomboid excision with Limberg flap reconstruction technique surely outscores elliptical excision with primary midline closure in certain important parameters. While facing a patient with uncomplicated sacrococcygeal pilonidal sinus surgeons should pose the question why not rhomboid excision with Limberg flap reconstruction instead of midline primary closure.

# 7. Marsupialization

Comparison between marsupialization, primary midline closure and flap technique for the treatment of pilonidal cyst was done by **Aycledett, E, et al**. from the Department of Surgery, Izmir Ataturk State Hospital (ANZ Surg 2001). They found that there was no difference in terms of wound infection or recurrence rates between the three groups, and the relatively shorter period of returning to work, emphasizes the usefulness of  excision and repair techniques in the surgical treatment of pilonidal disease.

# 8. Karydakis versus Limberg

**Bess A** from Alexandria University in Egypt compared short term results between the modified Karydakis and the modified Limberg flap (Dis.Colon Rectum 2013).

120 Patients with chronic pilonidal sinus disease were eligible for the study. Patients with sepsis were eligible only after aggressive treatment to eliminate sepsis.Operative time, postoperative complications,  patients  satisfaction with the cosmetic result, and the rate of recurrence were  studied, although the follow up times were not sufficient to evaluate long term recurrence rates.

His results were as follows : Of 154 patients screened, 125 were enrolled, and 120 patients completed the study.The median operative time was significantly shorter in patients with the modified Karydakis flap than those with the modified Limberg flap:33 (range 28-40) min vs 52 (range 48-62) min. No significant differences were found between  the study groups regarding overall complication rates , wound infection , subcutaneous fluid collection  or hyposthesia   . Full thickness wound disruption was encountered in 9 patients

(15%) in the modified Limberg group vs no patient in the modified Karydakis group . The median follow up duration was 20.5 months in each study group. One patient (2%) in the modified Karydakis group developed recurrent disease vs 2 patients (3%) in the modified Limberg group (p>0.99).In the modified Karydakis group  58 patients (97%) were satisfied with the cosmetic outcome and were  willing to recommend the operation to others vs 43 patients (72%) in the modified Limberg group (p<0.001).

**Conclusion: Both techniques provide effective treatment for pilonidal sinus** disease and can be performed safely as day case surgery. The modified Karydakis flap is associated with significantly shorter operative time, a lower full thickness wound disruption rate, and a higher patient satisfaction rate.

BUT AS THE AUTHORS MENTIONED IN THE BEGIN OF THEIR STUDY, THEY DID NOT ENROLL INFECTED CYST WITH ABSCESS FORMATION IN THE STUDY!

# 8. Karydakis / Bascom (with modifications)

The best description of the **Karydakis or Bascom technique** was given by Dr. Paul Kitchen, St. Vincent's Hospital,  Melbourne, who has followed the Karydakis method since seeing it performed by Karydakis himself in London 1973.

Dr. Kitchen describes it as follows :"He excised the sinus with a simple biconvex 'elliptical' excision only just crossing the midline to excise the sinus. It was based 1-2 cm from the midline with excision down to the sacrum. A thick flap was then created by undercutting the midline side of the wound. This flap was advanced  across the midline to meet the other side of the wound with two layers of catgut sutures to the fat around a drain tube. The wound was then closed with skin sutures"".

Karydakis believed and taught that hair insertion is the cause of pilonidal sinus and attributed his extremely low recurrence rate of 1% to two facts:

(a)  the whole wound is shifted away from the midline (recurrences always occur in the midline) and

(b)  the resulting new natal cleft is shallower (so hairs do not collect so readily).

Despite of these good results, the Karydakis operation has been criticized for taking too much fat, and for placing sutures into the midline sacral fascia (often causing pain).

Dr. Kitchen reports of 318 patients of whom 7(2%) had a recurrence requiring another procedure (curettage or a repeated Karydakis) and 5 (1%) had slight insignificant wound problems, easily dealt with simple measures without further surgery.

Dr. John Bascom in Oregon developed a similar operation which he called 'cleft lift'. It results in a similar, Karydakis- like looking wound off- midline, a shallow cleft . It is very successful in the treatment of difficult recurrent sinuses.

Several modifications have been proposed for Karydakis and Bascom procedures. Kitchen himself developed his own modification and  operates under local anaesthesia and intravenous sedation. The patients go home within 24 hours with less pain. No recurrences are seen so far.

# 9. Day-care surgery

**Abdul – Ghani AK et al.** from Whittington Hospital London suggest day care surgery for pilonidal sinus.

They operated 51 patient selectively as day care  surgery by excision and primary asymmetric closure.

They found that 4 weeks after operation 43 (88%) had complete healing and 6 (12%) had dehiscence of the wound. Recurrence rate was 8% (4 patients) after a follow up of 12-38 months. There was no admission from the day surgery unit and no unplanned re-admissions.

The cost for day-care pilonidal sinus surgery was estimated to be 672.00 pounds per patient compared with in patient cost of 2405.00 pounds.

**Conclusion**: Excision and primary asymmetric closure of pilonidal sinus is safe and feasible as day –care surgery and is associated with potential cost saving.

# 10. Other techniques

## Dufourmentel (1884-1957).

**Leon Dufourmentel,** born in France as a son of a merchant is remembered as the only practizing plastic surgeon in World War I.

During World War I he established a unit for maxillofacial surgery. In 1918 devised the graft technique named for him , Greffe Dufourmentel. He was the son–in-law of the anatomist Pierre Sebileau (1860-1953) and the father of the plastic surgeon Claude Dufourmentel (born 1915).

Leon Dufourmentel said in 1948, "If I went to Picasso for my portrait, he would probably make me a monster and I should be pleased because  it would be worth a million francs.But if Picasso came to me with a facial injury and I made him into a monster, aha, he might not be so pleased."

# **DUFOURMENTEL** and **LIMBERG**, BOTH MAXILLOFACIAL SURGEONS DEVELOPED NEARLY AT THE SAME TIME, MOST PROPABLY INDEPENDENT OF EACH OTHER, THE FLAP TECHNIQUE NAMED AFTER THEM ONE CENTURY BACK!!

The difference between the Limberg and the Dufourmentel flap are the angles. Although there is minimal difference, the Dufourmentel flap did not gain much publicity.

The first paper found was published 1991 in Dis Colon Rectum. No name mentioned, it reports about 25 patients operated between 1984-1989, 18 men and 7 women. No recurrence and no surgical wound infection occured.

A larger study appeared in Dis Colon rectum 2010, published by **Lieto E. Castellano P, Pinto M. et al**. , University of Naples Italy. The title of the study: **Dufourmentel rhomboid flap in the radical treatment of primary and recurrent sacrococcygeal pilonidal disease**.

The aim of the study was to assess early and late results of the Dufourmentel procedure in patients with primary and recurrent sacrococcygeal pilonidal disease.

All patients underwent epidural anesthesia and radical excision followed by reconstruction with a Dufourmentel rhomboid flap. Study variables included preoperative body mass index, hospital stay, time to walking, sitting and return to work, and pain score (visual analog scale) or evaluation early results and patient comfort. Time of complete wound healing, wound complications, and recurrence rates were recorded to assess late results.

**Results:** A total of 310 patients with pilonidal disease entered the study. Of these, 24 patients were asymptomatic (incidental diagnosis) and 55 had recurrent sinus. Obese patients had a significantly worse clinical presentation than patients with normal weight (P<.001). All operations were uneventful, with a mean operative time of 40 minutes. No flap necrosis occurred . The median hospital stay was 1 day(range 1-11 days), the median time of return to work was 7 (range 5-30) days, and pain was minimal. Wound complications were seen in 33 patients (10.6%). All but 2 patients were managed conservatively; in 2 patients (0.6%), the wound was resutured under local anesthesia and healed within 15 days. No patient was lost to follow up. Recurrence was observed in 7 patients (2.3%). All relapses occurred within 25 months after operation; no late recurrences were seen (5-,10-, and 16-year recurrence –free rates were all 97.6%). The recurrence rate was significantly higher in obese than in normal–weight patients (6% vs.0.5%; P=.0029). Permanent hypoesthesia was negligible (0.9%) and no patient complained about the cosmetic outcome.

**Conclusion: The Dufourmentel flap is associated with minimal discomfort and excellent results. This technique can be considered in the first and second line management of pilonidal disease.**

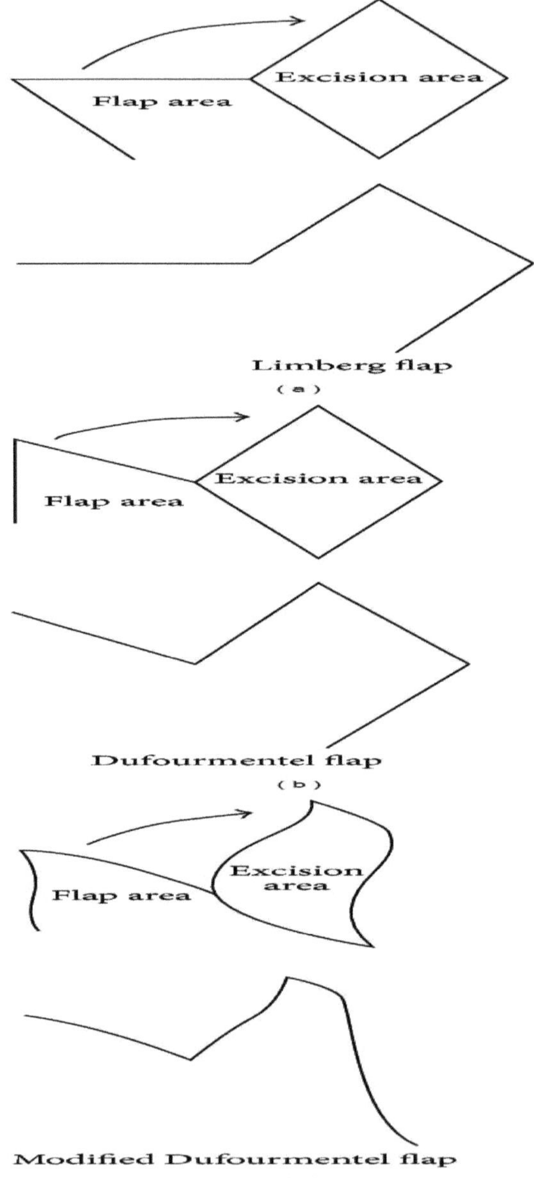


Limberg flap
( a )

Dufourmentel flap
( b )

Modified Dufourmentel flap
( c )

# 11. New techniques

## A. Bilateral gluteus maximus advancing flap

**A Comparison of the Limberg flap and bilateral gluteus advancing flap following oblique excision for the treatment of pilonidal sinus disease.**

Published by Yildar M, Cavdar F. in Surg Today 2013.

This study was performed to compare the use of a bilateral gluteus maximus advancing flap (BGMAF) following oblique incision, which was recently described for the surgical treatment of sacrococcygeal

**pilonidal sinus (SPS)** disease, with the widely used Limberg

flap(LF) technique following a rhomboid incision.

**Methods:** A total of 105 patients treated for SPS were evaluated retrospectively. The patients were evaluated in terms of their age, body mass index, symptoms, length of the operation, complications, postoperative hospital stay, time of return to work, postoperative cosmetic satisfaction and recurrence rate.

**Results:** Fifty six of the patients were treated with BGMAF, while 49 were treated with LF. The mean follow up was 20.5±5.4 months. The mean length of the operation, hospital stay and time to return to work were shorter, while the cosmetic satisfaction score was higher in the BGMAF group compared to the LF group. There was no statistically significant difference between the two groups for other criteria.

**Conclusion:** The BGMAF appears to be superior to the LF in terms of the length of the operation, time of return to work and degree of cosmetic satisfaction. It is preferable for sinuses which do not  require wide excision, while the LF is more appropriate for sinuses with a large post − excision defect.

# B. Video Assisted Treatment

**A video assisted ablation of pilonidal sinus: Newly minimally invasive treatment − A pilot study**

**Milone M, Musella M, et al**. from Naples Italy (Surgery 2013).

27 patients were operated with this technique. The authors found out that their results are encouraging and suggest that this technique may offer a very effective way to treat pilonidal sinus, but they also stated that further studies are necessary to validate its use in daily practice.

# C. Laser

Laser hair removal after surgery reduces the rate of recurrence by diminishing the number and thickness of hairs, as suggested by **Marzal** from London Clinic in Nurse Time 2013 .

He proposed to recommend it along with personal hygiene measures for patients to reduce short term and long term recuduction of recurrence.

# D. Vacuum Treatment

If the wound is left open after excision of pilonidal cyst VAC therapy might be considered (NPWT = negative pressure wound therapy).

But if the guidelines for the use of NPWT are not strictly followed, complication might occur. **Korean IJ , Sivrioghi S, Karacatt N**, from the Department of Plastic Surgery, Andan Menderes University, faculty of Medicine, Aydin, Turkey, published in J Wound Ostomy Continence Nurse 2013 a case of a 60 years old patient after excision of a pilonidal sinus which was managed after surgery with NPWT, unfortunately the patient developed squamous cell carcinoma.

# CONCLUSION:

As a conclusion concerning  all  treatment modalities of pilonidal cyst disease we can say that:

1. **There is still a large number of surgeons doing total excision with or without primary suturing. But they all agree that this method of treatment is accompanied by several complications. Therefore we can observe  a trend towards the flap repair.**

2. Among the flap repair techniques **the majority of  surgeons is using the Limberg flap**. Some are still using the Karydakis or Bascom technique with some modifications. There are no significant differences in results.

3. Some propose a slight **modification of the Limberg flap** by shifting the inferior incision off- midline (1-2 cm) so that there are no stitches in the midline. This modification is worth to be considered.

4. Surprisingly the **Dufourmentel flap is rarely used**, although only a little difference exists to the Limberg flap.

5. **The majority of the authors use the flap technique only in chronic pilonidal cyst disease**. We found no publications regarding the use of the Limberg flap in acute abscess formation. **There lays the main focus of our surgical strategy which will be discussed in the next chapter**.

6. As for the **video assisted excision** of pilonidal cyst, we think that this is not the proper place for such a minimally invasive procedure. Anyhow it is only at it's begin and needs enough feed back in the next years regarding recurrences and further complications.

7. The other "cosmetic" proposals **like laser hair removal** might be used in case of midline sutures and scars. They are of no use in case of flap repair.

8.Finally, there is unanimity that for

**extensive excision and large cavity**

**the Limberg flap remains the best**

**option.**

# PART III

# DEVELOPMENT OF OUR OWN TREATMENT CONCEPT.

In the United Arab Emirates pilonidal cyst is a relatively frequent disease  due to climatic conditions and the stronger trunk hairiness of many of the nationalities who are present here. Because of the given working conditions, where in case of an illness everyone is afraid to loose his job,nearly all our patients with pilonidal cysts come at the stage of abscess-formation for treatment, and endeavour to resume work as soon as possible. In order to meet this difficult situation surgically, we had to make a virtue of necessity. We have **abandoned the prevalent doctrin thatprimary Limberg plasty is only applicable in non-infected pilonidal cysts!**

**OUR OWN TREATMENT STRATEGY.**

Since 2006 we use the Limberg plasty without exception as primary definitive treatment also in **abscess-forming or chronic fistulating pilonidal cysts.**

Only if the abscess has spread to neighbouring gluteal area, and cannot be excised completely because of large tissue loss, we do **open treatment** with **secondary Limberg repair** as soon the excision wound is clean and shows good granulation tissue (on average after 2 weeks).

**Technique of Limberg rotation-flap_repair**

Picture 1

Picture 2

Marking of the lines for rhomboid excision of the pilonidal cyst and the Limberg flap (either left or right, depending on the main side of the abscess).The lateral length of the rhombus and the rotation-flap is 4-5 cm on average (up to 7 cm!).

Picture 3

After injection of Methylen-blue dye into the fistula or the abscess in order to mark the borders, the pilonidal cyst is excised completely along the drawing lines, down to the presacral fascia. Meticulous hemostasis by cautery.

Picture 4

Cyst is excised, the rotation-flap is circumcised and separated from the muscular fascia.

Picture 5

Insertion of Redivac drain and hemostyptic Lyostypt-foam, soaked with Gentamycin)

Picture 6

The flap is rotated into the defect and fixed with 4/0 Prolene mattress-sutures

Picture 7

Rotation-flap sutured

Picture 8

Late result of Limberg-flap repair

## PILONIDAL – SURGERY at CEDARS 9/2004 - 12/2013:

**121 cases** (117 male, 4 female patients)

9/2004 – 5/2006: Excision with open treatment (12 cases)

6/2006 – 2/2013: Excision with Limberg-  flap repair (109 cases)

Only 4 of the 109 cases presented with an **asymptomatic pilonidal sinus** (just midline pits in the presacral area), whereas 105 were **pilonidal abscesses** or **chronic-fistulating pilonidal cysts.**

---

## <u>Surgical procedures:</u>

**2006 - 2013**

•Excision & primary Limberg rotation-flap repair: **101** cases

•Excision & secondary Limberg rotation-flap repair: **8 cases**

---

## Postoperative treatment & course

•Hospital stay 2 days

•Redivac-drain for 48 hours

•Antibiotic treatment for 7 days (Amoxycillin + Clavulan acid)

•Suture removal after 14 days

•Normal lifestyle after 4 days (shower)

•Return to work on average after 14 days

---

## Results:

•3 cases of superficial infection with delayed healing

•No hematomas or seromas

•No flap-necrosis (not even partial!)

•Minimal postoperative pain

•No recurrences until now (1-90 months)

•Numbness of the flap not reported

•Good satisfaction with the cosmetic result

**SUMMARY**

•We have established a **standardized, extremely successful treatment strategy** of **pilonidal disease** at our hospital.

•**Limberg plasty** is a technically easy and definitive treatment for **all categories** of pilonidal cysts.

•This procedure guarantees excellent results with high **satisfaction** of **patient & surgeon!**

# CONCLUSION AND MESSAGE

The general application of the Limberg plasty in every course of pilonidal disease to our surprise has proven to us as a **"foolproof" surgical procedure**, which can be recommended without reservation as worth emulating.

It guarantees high treatment satisfaction for the patient as well as for the surgeon, since they have not to go through a frustrating open wound treatment for weeks.

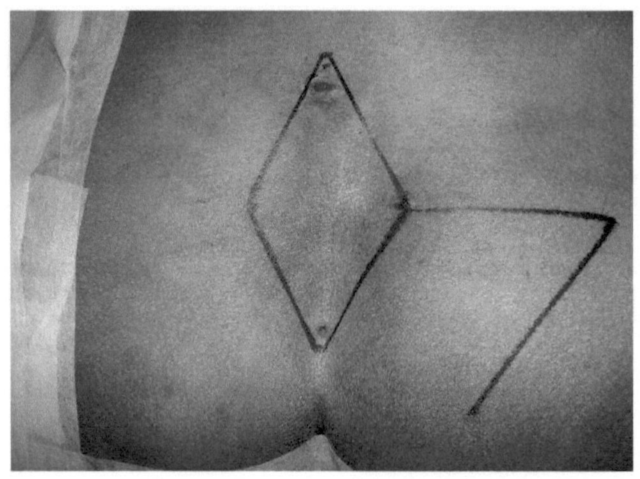

**Picture 1**

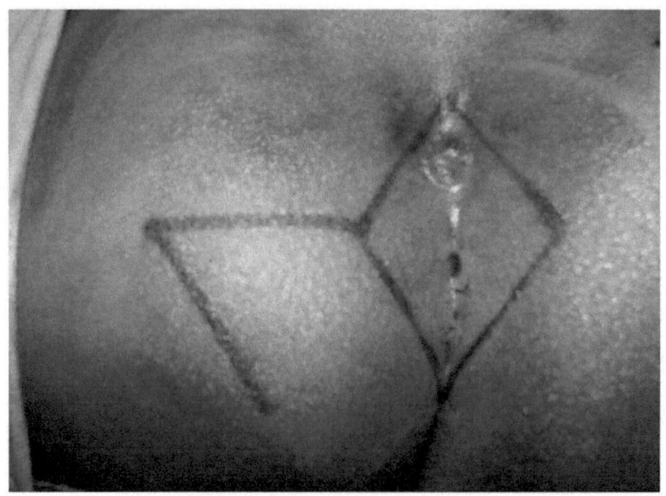

**Picture 2**

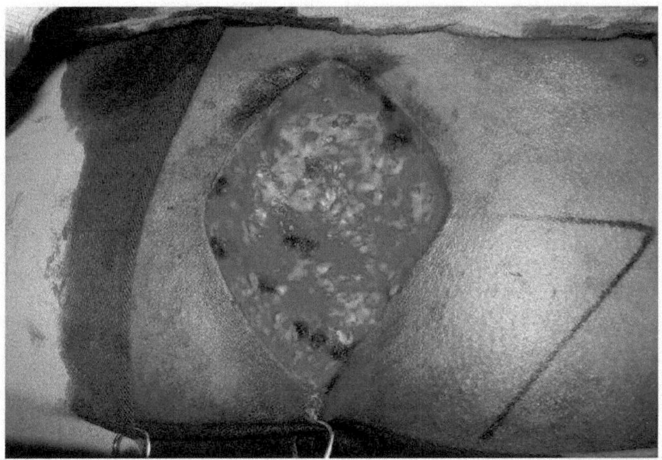

**Picture 3**

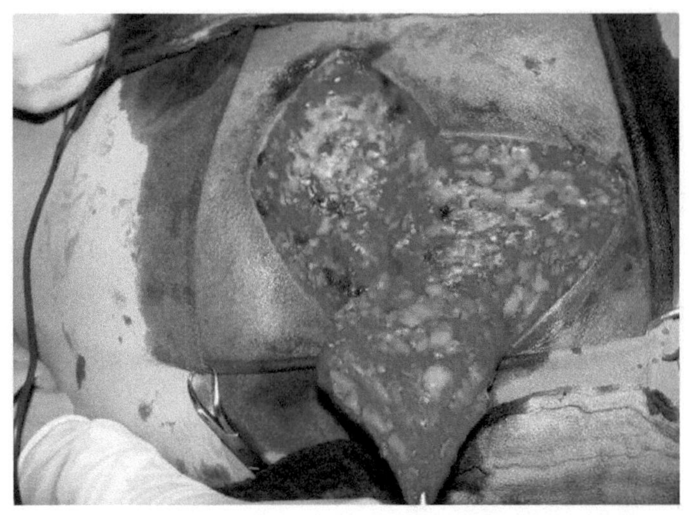

**Picture 4**

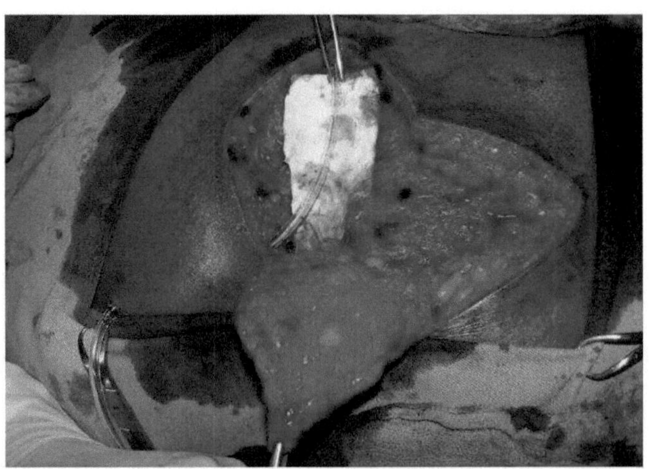

**Picture 5**

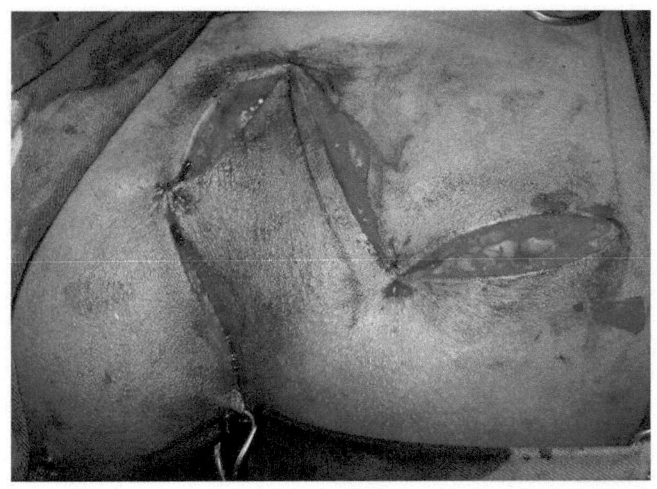

**Picture 6**

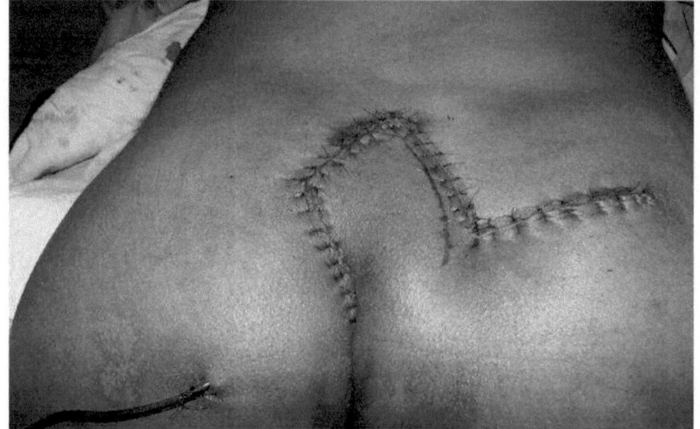

**Picture 7**

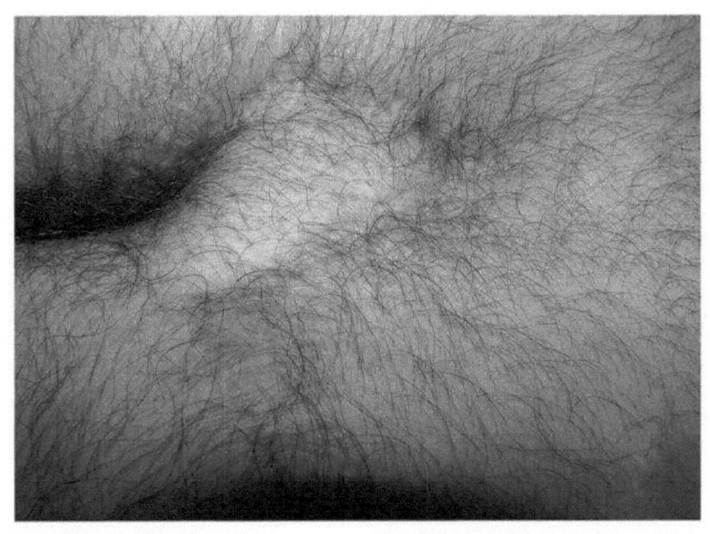

**Picture 8**

**Same approach on right side with intracutaneous suturing:**

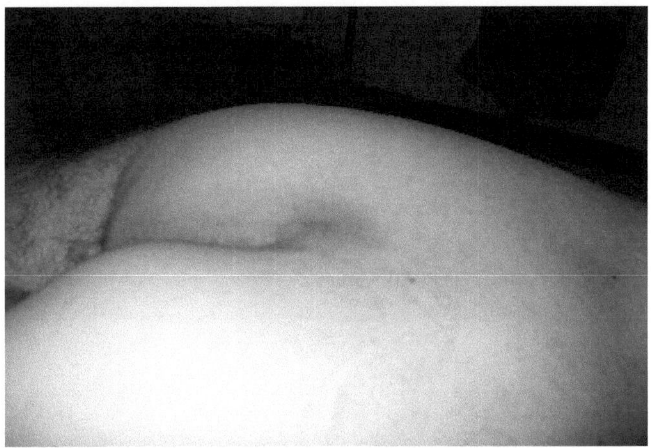

**Picture 9**

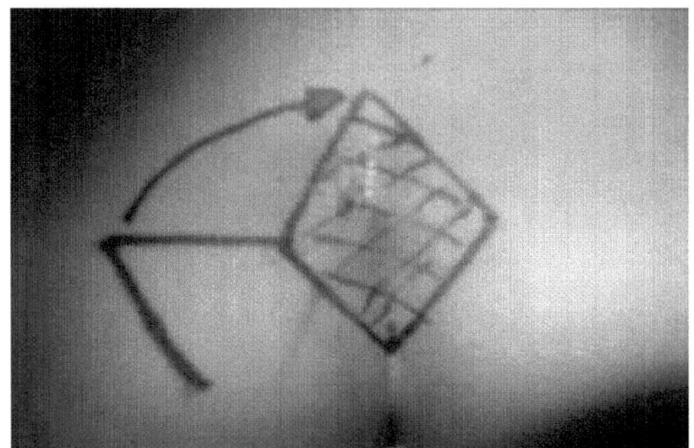

**Picture 10**

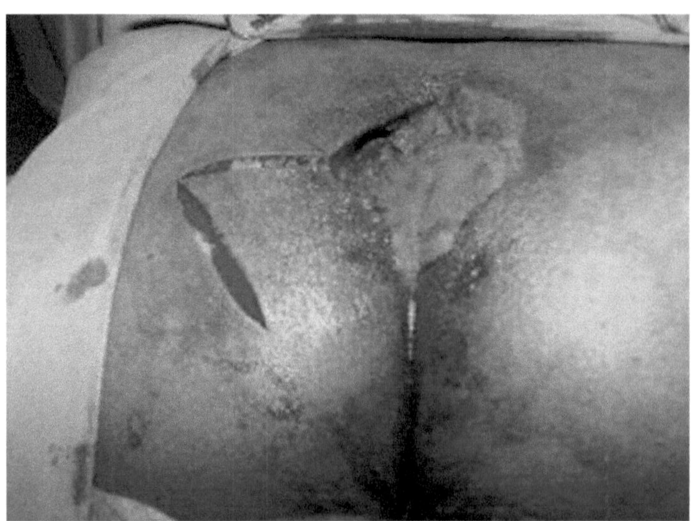

**Picture 11**

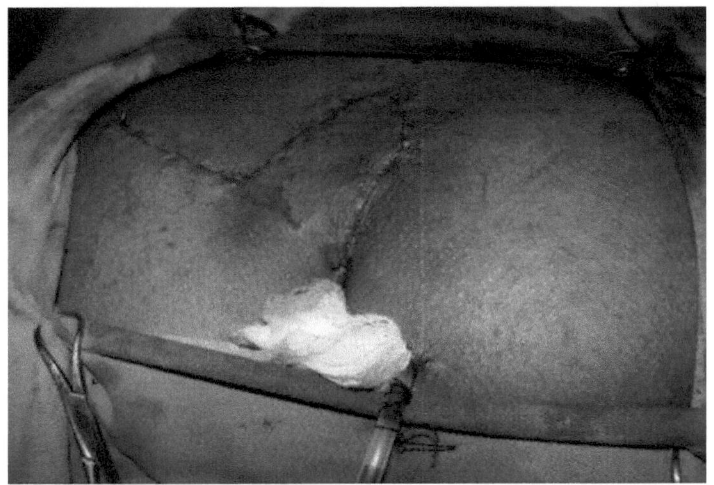

**Picture 12**

# TABLE OF CONTENTS

**REFERENCES**


1.      Mentes BB, Leventoglu S, Cihan A, Tatlicioglu E, Akin M, Oguz M. Modified Limberg transposition flap for sacrococcygeal pilonidal sinus. Surg Today. 2004;34(5):419-23.


2.      Ozgültekin R, Ersan Y, Ozcan M, Ozçelik F, Celik V, Cerçel A, Sakaoğlu M. Therapy of pilonidal sinus with the Limberg transposition flap. Chirurg. 1995 Mar; 66(3):192-5.


3.      Topgül K, Ozdemir E, Kiliç K, Gökbayir H, Ferahköşe Z. Long-term results of limberg flap procedure for treatment of pilonidal sinus: a report of 200 cases. Dis Colon Rectum. 2003 Nov;46(11):1545-8.


4.      Akin M, Gokbayir H, Kilic K, Topgul K, Ozdemir E, Ferahkose Z. Rhomboid excision and Limberg flap for managing pilonidal sinus: long-term results in 411 patients. Colorectal Dis. 2008 Nov;10(9):945-8. Epub 2008 May 3.


5.      Mentes O, Bagci M, Bilgin T, Ozgul O, Ozdemir M. Limberg flap procedure for pilonidal sinus disease: results of 353 patients. Langenbecks Arch Surg. 2008 Mar;393(2):185-9. Epub 2007 Sep 22.


6.      Akca T, Colak T, Ustunsoy B, Kanik A, Aydin S. Randomized clinical trial comparing primary closure with the Limberg flap in the treatment of primary sacrococcygeal pilonidal disease. Br J Surg. 2005 Sep;92(9):1081-4.

7.      Azab AS, Kamal MS, Saad RA, Abou al Atta KA, Ali NA. Radical cure of pilonidal sinus by a transposition rhomboid flap. Br J Surg. 1984 Feb;71(2):154-5.

8.      B. R. Gwynn. Use of the rhomboid flap in pilonidal sinus. Ann R Coll Surg Engl. 1986 January; 68(1): 40–41.

9.      T. Holmebakk, A. Nesbakken. Surgery for Pilonidal Disease. Scandinavian Journeal of Surgery 94:43-46, 2005

10.     Eryilmaz R, Sahin M, Alimoglu O, Dasiran F. Surgical treatment of sacrococcygeal pilonidal sinus with the Limberg transposition flap. Surgery. 2003 Nov;134(5):745-9.

11.     Azab AS, Kamal MS, Saad RA, Abou al Atta KA, Ali NA. Radical cure of pilonidal sinus by a transposition rhomboid flap. Br J Surg. 1984 Feb;71(2):154-5.

12.     Jaschke CW, Mährlein R, Mangold G. [Results of the Limberg transposition flap in the treatment of pilonidal sinus] Zentralbl Chir. 2002 Aug;127(8):712-5.

13.     Arumugam PJ, Chandrasekaran TV, Morgan AR, Beynon J, Carr ND. The rhomboid flap for pilonidal disease. Colorectal Dis. 2003 May;5(3):218-21.

14.     Cihan A, Mentes BB, Tatlicioglu E, Ozmen S, Leventoglu S, Ucan BH. Modified Limberg flap reconstruction compares favourably with primary repair for pilonidal sinus surgery. ANZ J Surg. 2004 Apr;74(4):238-42.

15.     Urhan MK, Kücükel F, Topgul K, Ozer I, Sari S. Rhomboid excision and Limberg flap for managing pilonidal sinus: results of 102 cases. Dis Colon Rectum. 2002 May;45(5):656-9.

16.     Misiakos EP, Troupis T, Hatzikokolis S, Macheras A, Liakakos T, Patapis P, Karatzas G. Limberg flap reconstruction for the treatment of pilonidal sinus disease. Chirurgia (Bucur). 2006 Sep-Oct;101(5):513-7

17.     Bozkurt MK, Tezel E. Management of pilonidal sinus with the Limberg flap. Dis Colon Rectum. 1998 Jun;41(6):775-7.

18.     El-Khadrawy O, Hashish M, Ismail K, Shalaby H. Outcome of the rhomboid flap for recurrent pilonidal disease. World J Surg. 2009 May;33(5):1064-8.

19.     Deya M Marzouk,[1] Ahmed A Abou-Zeid,[2] Anthony Antoniou,[1] Amyn Haji,[1] and H Benziger[1].Sinus Excision, Release of Coccycutaneous Attachments and Dermal-Subcuticular Closure (XRD Procedure): A Novel Technique in Flattening the Natal Cleft in Pilonidal Sinus Treatment. Ann R Coll Surg Engl. 2008 July; 90(5): 371–376.

20.     Buie LA. Jeep disease (pilonidal disease of merchanized warfare). South Medications J 1944; 37:103.

21.     Karydakis GE. Easy and successful treatmet of piloindal sinus after explanation of its causative process. Aust N Z J Surg 1992; 62:385-9.

22.     Bascom J, Bascom T. Utility of the cleft lift procedure in refractory pilonidal disease. Am J Surg 2007;193:606-609.

23.     Kitchen PRB. Pilonidal sinus: experience with the Karydakis flap. Br J Surg 1996;83:1452-5.

24.     Arumugam Pj et al. The rhomboid flap for pilonidal disease. Colorectal Dis. 2003; 5:218-21.

25.    Postoperative patients' characteristics after follow-up. Indian J Plast Surg. 2009 Jan–Jun; 42(1): 43–48.


26.    Ann R Coll Surg Engl.2006 Nov; 88(7):656-8. Day –care surgery for pilonidal sinus. Abdul-Ghani AK, Abdul-Ghani AN, Ingham Clark CL. Department of Surgery, Whittington Hospital, London, UK.


27.    ANZ J. Surg.2001 Jun; 71 (6):362- 4. Comparison of three methods in surgical treatment of pilonidal disease. Aydede H, Erhan Y, Sakarya A, Kumkumoglu Y.


28.    Colorectal Dis.2012 Feb;14(2): 143-51.doi:10.1111/j. 1463 -1318. 2010.024736.x. Primary closure or rhomboid excision and Limberg flap for the management of primary sacrococcygeal pilonidal disease? A meta-analysis of randomized controlled trials. Horwood J, Hanratty D, Chandran P, Billings P.


29. BMJ. 2008 Apr 19; 336 (7659):868 – 71. doi:10.1136/bmj.39517.808160.BE.Epub 2008 Apr7. Healing by primary closure versus open healing after surgery for pilonidal sinus: systematic review and meta-analysis. Mc.Callum IJ, King PM, Bruce J.


30. Can J Plast Surg 2007; 15(2):67-71.The versatile rhomboid (Limberg) flap. Leslie R Chasmar, MD FRCSC


31. http://www.emedicinehealth.com/pilonidal_cyst/page9_em.htm


32. http://www.emedicinehealth.com/pilonidal_cyst/page7_em.htm


33. http://www.emedicinehealth.com/pilonidal_cyst/page8_em.htm


34. http://www.emedicinehealth.com/pilonidal_cyst/page6_em.htm


35. http://www.emedicinehealth.com/pilonidal_cyst/page3_em.htm

36. http://www.emedicinehealth.com/pilonidal_cyst/page2_em.htm


37. http://www.emedicinehealth.com/pilonidal_cyst/article_em.htm


38. Br J Hosp Med (Lond). 2010 Sep; 71 (9):511-3. The Limberg flap in sacrococcygeal pilonidal sinus disease. Shetty R, Payne R.


39. Dis Colon Rectum 2004 Feb;47(2);233-7. Limberg flap repair for pilonidal sinus disease. Daphan C, Tekelioglu MH, Sayilgan C. Department of General Surgery, University of Kirikkale School of Medicine, Kirikkale, Turkey.
cagatayereden@hotmail.com


40. J Pak Med Assoc. 2009 Mar; 59 (3):157-60. Open excision with secondary healing versus rhomboid excision with Limberg transposition flap in the management of sacrococcygeal pilonidal disease. Jamal A, Shamim M, Hashmi F, Qureshi MI.
Surgical Unit IV, Liaquat University Hospital, Jamshoro, Pakistan.


41. Surg Today, 2004; 34(5):419-23. Modified Limberg transposition flap for sacrococcygeal pilonidal sinus. Mentes BB, Leventoglu S, Cihan A, Tatlicioglu E,
Akin M, Oguz M.


42. J Eur Acad Dermatol Venereol. 2010 Jan; 24(1): 7-12. doi:10.1111/j.1468-3083.2009.03350.x, Epub 2009 Jul 13. Surgical treatment of sacrococcygeal pilonidal sinus with rhomboid flap. Topgul K. Department of Surgery, School of Medicine, Ondukoz Mayis University, Samsun, Turkey.ktopgul@gmail.com


43. J Korean Surg Soc 2013 August; 85(2):63-67. Published online 2013 July 25. doi:10.4174/jkss.2013.58.2.63. Comparison of the limberg flap with the V-Y flap technique in the treatment of pilonidal disease. Fatih Altintoprak, [1] Enis Dickicier,
[2] Yusuf Arslan, [2] Taner Ozkececi, [3] Gokhan Akbulut,[1,3] and Osman Nuri Dilek[1]

44.Indian J surg.2012 August;749(4):305-308 Published online 2012 January 7. doi 10.1007/s12262-011-0400-9. Elliptical Excision with Midline Primary Closure Versus Rhomboid Excision with Limberg flap Reconstruction in Sacrococcygeal Pilonidal Disease: A Prospective, Randomized Study. Tufale A. Dass, [1] Muneer Zaz, [1] Ajaz Rather,[2] and Shamsul Bari [2]

45.Scientific World Journal.2013; 2013:807027. Published online 2013 May 14. doi 10.1155/2013/807027. Karydakis Flap Procedure in Patients with Sacrococcygeal Pilonidal Sinus Disease: Experience of a Single Centre in Istanbul. M. Kamil Yildiz, Erkan Ozkan, Haci Mehmet Odabasi, Bulent Kaya, Cengiz Eris, Haci Hassan Abouglu, Emre Gunay, Mehmet M, Fersahoglu and Suleyman Atalay.

46. Br Med J.1953 April 25; 1(4816):936,937. Pilonidal Sinus of the Suprapubic region A.R. Currie, Thomas Gibson and Archd L. Goodall

47. Abu Galala KH, Salam IMA, Abu Samaan KR et al.: Treatment of pilonidal sinus by primary closure with a transported rhomboid flap compared with deep suturing: a prospective randomized clinical trial. Eur. J Surg.165 (1999) 468 – 472.

48. Akca T, Colak T, Ustonsoy B et al.: Randomized clinical trial comparing primary closure with the Limberg flap.

49. Bascom J: Pilonidal disease: long term results of follicle removal. Dis Colon Rectum 12 (1983) 800 – 807.

50. Davis KA, Mock CN, Versaci A et al.: Malignant degeneration of pilonidal cysts. Am. Surg.60 (1994)200-204.

51. Duxbury MS, Blake SM, Dashfield A et al.:A randomized trial of knife versus diathermy in pilonidal disease. Ann. R. Coll. Surg.Engl. 85(2003) 405-407.

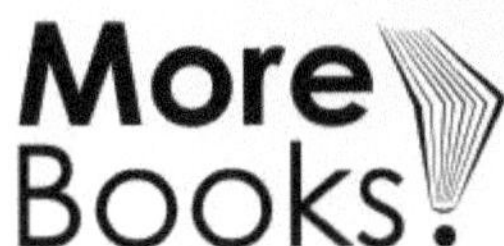


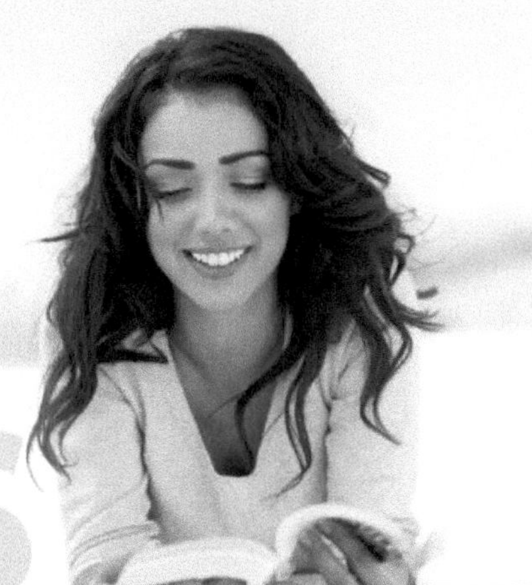



Buy your books fast and straightforward online - at one of world's fastest growing online book stores! Environmentally sound due to Print-on-Demand technologies.

Buy your books online at
**www.morebooks.shop**

Kaufen Sie Ihre Bücher schnell und unkompliziert online – auf einer der am schnellsten wachsenden Buchhandelsplattformen weltweit! Dank Print-On-Demand umwelt- und ressourcenschonend produzi ert.

Bücher schneller online kaufen
**www.morebooks.shop**

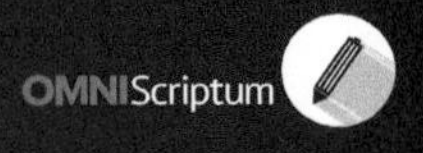

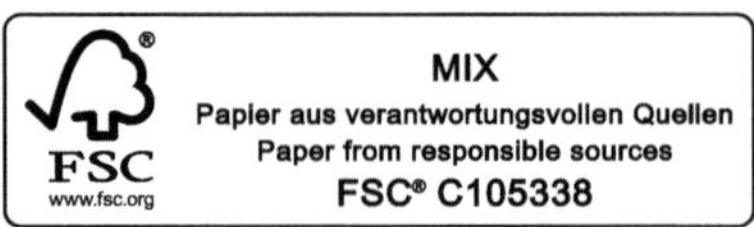


Printed by Books on Demand GmbH, Norderstedt / Germany